Exercise with Ehlers Danlos Syndrome

Claire Hunter

Exercise with Ehlers Danlos Syndrome
First Edition

ISBN: 978-1-71684-883-4

Safety note.

It is important to seek medical advice before beginning any kind of exercise programme.

The advice in this book is generalised for otherwise healthy individuals with Hypermobility Spectrum Disorders. Comorbidities such as POTS and fibromyalgia, or your unique anatomy should be taken into consideration.

Always see your doctor if you are injured or rehabilitating from an injury.

Seek a knowledgeable fitness professional who can assess your suitability for a new programme and support you in learning how to move well.

The information in this book is aimed at people with Hypermobility Spectrum Disorder who have been cleared by their GP to exercise. There are times that I use EDS or HSD interchangeably, this is a linguistic attempt to use the older, more commonly used terminology for comfort, while acknowledging recent understanding of Hypermobility disorders as a spectrum. If you have hypermobile joints with a decreased ability to access mainstream exercise - I'm talking to you. I may reference other symptoms that are common in people with HSD, if this is not relevant to you, please feel free to disregard that point.

Why are we here?

Exercise and EDS have a complex relationship.

When I was first diagnosed I was told not to exercise by some doctors, and encouraged to by others. One doctor told me I should dose up on ibuprofen and compete in cross country running, another told me that doing so would leave me unable to walk without aid before I was 20. My physiotherapist gave me strength exercises, but other EDS specialists said to just be active. It was a minefield, and it still is.

I spend a lot of time on hypermobility support groups, and I hear a lot of advice.

"Don't run, it will ruin your knees"
"Don't do yoga, it will make you stretchier"
"Don't wear supports, it will weaken your muscles"

And the opposite always comes up too. No one is really sure.

Who am I and why do I get a say?

Hi! I'm Claire, I am a zebra. I have EDS, with features of Classical and Hypermobility type, I also have fibromyalgia and autonomic dysfunction.

I am an athlete, I'm a competitive powerlifter, I can run, although I prefer not to, I'm also a dancer and I love yoga. This wasn't always the case, I spent most of my twenties with moderate mobility issues and kinesiophobia.

Which is why I ended up as a Personal Trainer. I'm also a Corrective Exercise Specialist, which means I work with people who have chronic joint misalignment and movement dysfunction (often due to old injuries, occupational habits or.…hypermobility) that causes them pain, repetitive injury or impaired performance. And I sort that right out.

I'm not a doctor, or a physiotherapist, which means I won't diagnose problems or attempt to treat injuries or ill health. My job is preventing future injuries, training healthy movement and removing the barriers that stop people from being able to access a healthy lifestyle - sometimes this is physical, sometimes psychological.

What is this book for?

My aim with this book is to un-muddy the waters surrounding exercising with EDS.

I find myself answering the same questions over and over, which tells me that there is a need for a simple primer to help people with hypermobility take their first steps into an exercise programme.

We are going to explore some of the commonly held beliefs about EDS and exercise, and do a bit of mythbusting.

I'm going to give you some information that should help you decide what steps you need to take.

And I am also providing you with a basic introductory programme to get you started.

I've tried to keep things as concise as possible, so you can get your teeth into the programme as smoothly as possible. If you would like more in-depth information, I am happy to take questions (my contact information is at www.firelotusfitness.com) or my blog, linked from the same site, has articles under the EDS label. I've included edited versions of a couple of the most relevant articles, in Part 3 of this book.

Part 1 - To exercise, or not to exercise?

Why exercising with EDS seems like a bad idea

If you are diagnosed with a Hypermobility Spectrum Disorder (HSD) it is likely that this happened after pain or injury. People who don't have pain or injury tend not to seek medical help, let alone pursue it to the point of a specialist diagnosis.

So you started the journey with a fresh injury, and it was likely the first thing you were told was to rest and heal - entirely legitimate. Your body reacts to injury in a number of ways, and many of them have the function of preventing you from using the injured area - so it can heal. That was your first priority.

Over time, people with HMS tend to suffer repetitive injuries. Hypermobile joints are unstable and prone to dislocation, subluxation and sprains. The laxity in your connective tissue affects your proprioception (your ability to sense where your body is in space). This makes you clumsy and accident prone. Overall,you spend a lot of time resting injuries and gain a sense that maybe an activity that risks injury isn't a good plan.

Your body is totally in on this too. When you are injured, your nervous system adapts to protect the injured area. Muscles tighten into spasm, to create stability, the signals to other muscles are dulled, so they become underactive, reducing strength and range of motion. Last of all your nervous system creates the sensation of pain - a warning to prevent further injury.

Hang on a minute, did I just say our nervous system creates pain?

I absolutely did, pain is an output from the nervous system, it is generated to keep us safe. Which means that it can be generated when there is no input (like an injury) from the body. That's why "old injuries" that appear physically healed can continue to give us pain and stiffness for years afterwards - the nervous system is still trying to protect the area, like a fire alarm sounding long after the burnt toast has been thrown out.

As your body finds workarounds to avoid the painful or tight areas, your movement patterns become compromised, making you even more prone to injury and the cycle continues.

One of the biggest barriers to exercise in people with chronic pain or fatigue is kinesiophobia. This is the fear that exercise may make symptoms worse, or lead to injury.

It is a valid concern that is reinforced when someone with a chronic condition attempts an exercise programme or activity which is inappropriate to their needs and becomes ill or injured as a result. It can be very hard to trust someone who is encouraging you to exercise, knowing that the last attempt ended badly.

Why people with EDS should exercise

Everyone should be exercising! Absolutely everyone who is remotely able.

That might sound a bit fervent, but it's absolutely true. Our bodies function better on exercise. Cardiovascular health, absolutely key to being alive for a reasonable amount of time - improved by exercise. Bone health, metabolism, organ function, preventing decline of health with age…. exercise.

Cardio is good, resistance training is good, mobility is good. Exercise is brilliant!

In hypermobile bodies, there are a number of key benefits of exercise.

Cardiovascular exercise
- increases stamina
- reduces fatigue
- improves the efficiency of your energy systems
- releases endorphins to counter chronic pain

Resistance training (building strength and muscle mass)
- creates stability around joints
- increases strength in connective tissue
- trains healthy movement patterns
- restores mind-muscle connection

Mobility work (working on range of motion and control)
- releases overactive (tightened) areas
- trains healthy movement patterns and range of motion
- improves body awareness and proprioception

It is quite clear that exercise is a necessary component if our goal is to live a healthy life with HSD. It can both improve overall health and help manage symptoms. Yet starting exercise is a tricky path to navigate well.

How should people with EDS exercise?

Whenever anyone asks me what the best exercise is, my classic response is this:

The best exercise for you is any activity that you can safely enjoy and consistently incorporate into your life.

I could write the perfect programme, carefully structured to take into account every idiosyncrasy in your unique body. Perfectly safe, balanced between cardio and resistance. Well managed recovery, exemplary nutrition....

But it would only work if you were able to follow it, long term.

That's the tough part. I suspect like me, you have been to a physiotherapist at some point and been given exercises to do 3 times a day, and you probably didn't last longer than a week. That's OK, no one is judging you, it's quite usual and the experts on physical therapy for EDS now recognise that completing some kind of activity is far more effective than avoiding the "perfect" programme.

So what's your aspiration?

How would you like to incorporate exercise and activity into your life? If you're reading this, you likely have something in mind, a sport you used to play but can't currently access perhaps? Or are you a cycling nut waiting to break out? Maybe you are a hiker, or a dancer? Or you fancy joining your work mates for Zumba class.

You might not be ready to start on it yet, but knowing where you want to go will help your motivation now.

There are people with HMS out there running marathons (whoops, that's the no running concept out of the window), competing in CrossFit, Gymnastics, all sorts. Don't make the mistake of thinking this is a reflection of the severity of their condition, the right training and management can lead to incredible results.

The mistake people make is trying to get there too fast. Every body needs to be prepared for athletic endeavours, our bodies need a bit more care.

More modest aspirations are of course welcome, I offer the above examples as an extreme, but if your long term exercise goal is to maintain your allotment, walk your dog regularly or cycle to work, that's brilliant. Hold on to it.

Exercise to avoid, or not

You might guess from the above that there really isn't a one size fits all dos and don'ts list, but there are some things that I would approach with caution, and not recommend to those new or returning to exercise with HSD

Impact/plyometrics

Jumping, running, anything that has a heavy impact on the joints needs to be approached with caution at the outset.

In a good, progressive exercise programme, no plyometric work should be included until after phases of corrective exercise, stability and strength building - it's just not entry level stuff. For anyone.

Sometimes general population exercise classes will include this type of thing to "make it interesting", but anyone starting out shouldn't be pushing themselves.

I have observed that people with EDS often build muscle strength fast, but connective tissue strength more slowly. This means that you might be powerful enough to make a box jump, but not stable enough within your joints to land it without injury. HSD athletes need to spend longer in the muscular strength phase of their programme.

I've included running under this banner. Lots of people with HSD are able to run. However most people with HSD starting out at exercise will have a dysfunctional gait. In other words it's not so much the running that is the issue, but that running highlights existing problems in the body.

I recommend starting with walking and strength work to stabilise and correctly align the body. Once that is achieved then running in a healthy gait is achievable.

We tend to assume that we "know" how to run, but having observed many people both on the treadmill and out in the wild, I can assure you that very few people run, or walk very well without a little correction! The good news, if you are an aspiring runner, is that there is a lot of good information available to help you with the basics, and a coach can help you from there.

Stretching

Well, here is a contentious issue.

It's often assumed that as we are "too flexible" that stretching will make us worse due to it making us "more flexible".

This makes absolute sense. It's also not at all correct.

You see, in the vast majority of situations stretching does not change the length of the muscle fibres or connective tissue. You don't make your muscles longer by stretching them. If you did, they would get too long for your bones and you would fall down like a marionette.

In HSD the connective tissue is more elastic, not too long. And stretching doesn't increase elasticity either.

What stretching actually does is stimulate the nervous system to release the muscle. So if a muscle is slightly contracted and reducing the range of motion, stretching can signal to the brain to release the muscle and restore the correct range of motion.

[progressive stretching does exist, in ballet dancers and gymnasts for instance, chronic programmes of prolonged stretching are used to encourage flexibility, but this is always in conjunction with strength work and is not applicable to general fitness programming.]

It is likely that anyone with hypermobility, and the associated history of injury and instability, will have overactive muscles that would benefit from release in order to restore the range of motion necessary for healthy movement within a joint.

For example, if your ankles roll in and your feet flatten, the lateral (outside) calf is probably tight. Your ankle won't move correctly until balance is restored.

Failing to release these areas leads to injury at the directly affected joint, or compensation somewhere else in the body. For instance, that ankle roll can be compensated for by inward rotation of the thigh (leading to a knock-kneed posture) which translates to a forward tilted pelvis which means…. lower back pain.

If that all seems a bit deep, don't worry, just trust me on the stretching.

I prefer to programme dynamic stretching that explores the range of motion under control. I avoid forcing a stretch past the point of comfort. I also use myofascial release to encourage the release of overactive muscle without stretching.

While it might seem like good sense to "lock down" all your unstable joints, if you want functional movement, you need to have freedom to move.

Complex coordination

If your activity requires you to move in complicated ways, to activate multiple muscle groups together or to mentally process several things at once - consider that something to work towards. It's not a starting point.

If you are running around a squash court or negotiating long circuits of complicated HIIT exercises, you won't have the capacity to ensure that you are moving healthily all the time. It's easy to fudge a movement and roll an ankle or twist a knee.

We build up to this sort of exercise by first strengthening muscles and practicing beautiful movement patterns.

Intensity vs endurance

Another way to lose focus and slip into sloppy movement is to be tired.

At the end of a long run, or a long set of strength exercises, fatigue is liable to trip you up.

Similarly, if you are pushing at your absolute hardest, your form is going to fail.

We aim for the sweet spot of about 80%. We stop before we have to. We make every movement good, so that our bodies learn to always move well.

Part 2 - Getting into exercise - from couch to capable

A healthy person with well managed EDS and an understanding of their unique capabilities and needs should be able to access beginner level fitness classes or standard fitness programmes.

I would recommend aiming for small-group settings with plenty of coaching and feedback from a knowledgeable instructor.

But that information is only useful if you are fit enough to access those options. Many people who have been living with EDS for a long while have movement issues that need addressing first, or are not fit enough to "keep up" in a generalised setting without causing themselves harm.

Never fear! This is what this section is for!

I'm going to give you a starting programme that assumes only that you can walk, on the flat, for 10 minutes at a time, at your own pace. The goal of this is to improve your joint stability, strength and movement capability so that you can step up onto the first rung towards your aspirational exercise.

Some individuals with EDS may still have issues accessing this generalised programme. I work one to one with those with more limited mobility, or a need for a specialised corrective programme and if this is you, please do seek support.

I have not included a corrective phase in this programme, as this is an individual process that requires assessment, however the stability phase includes elements to improve some basic corrective work.

Before we start

Let's get ourselves set up for success.

Routine

You're going to be training for 3 sessions a week. Ideally you will not train on consecutive days, because recovery is super important. Monday, Wednesday, Friday is ideal. If you have to do 2 days in a row, that's OK, but never 3 - that's madness.

Set your day and time, and stick with it. Put it in your diary and commit to it. Now is a good time to build a habit, so maybe put it in the slot where that class you have your eye on falls.

Mindset

Feeling a bit tentative? That's normal.

Making changes is always tough. What if it doesn't work? What if it does? Either outcome has its own set of anxieties associate with it.

Set yourself up for success by trying these tips:

Schedule

Decide when you are going to train, put it in the diary, put an alarm on your phone. That's your slot. Stick to it. It's easier to discipline ourselves to stick with a new regime when we make the decisions in advance.

Recognise that you are safe

This programme is designed for people like you. It is about gently introducing your body to safe movement. "No pain, no gain" doesn't belong here. Your school PE teacher who accused you of faking isn't here. You are in control while you are learning more about working with your body.

It's OK to make adjustments if you need to (the instruction videos cover some scaling and you are welcome to contact me for alternatives). It's also OK to decide not to train today, if you are unwell. The question to ask yourself is "will this workout leave me feeling better, or worse". If the former, it's time to put your getting-things-done pants on, if the latter, maybe just do the mobility session and a gentle stroll instead (but try and do something in your scheduled slot to honour the habit).

Prioritise your health

I suggest putting your workout in your diary for a second reason, it stops you from deprioritising it if something else comes up. You're not available at that time, just as you wouldn't be available if you had a dentist appointment.

Focus on your goals

I said earlier that the best exercise was whatever you enjoyed doing consistently. But I know that for some people an introductory programme isn't that thing.

Remember that this is just the first step of the process. Your goal here is to build the strength, balance and stability to start to do more things that you really enjoy. Keep your eye on the prize and keep going. This part is transient.

Make it easy to get into

Keep your workout clothes handy, keep your space tidy, make it simple to just get in there and get on with it, no fussing.

Enjoy your workouts

Try to make your workout space fun to be in, demand space and privacy. Play music you enjoy, try different kinds. Maybe you'll like working out to bouncy energetic music, or cheerful upbeat music, or angry powerful music. I have found that I really like doing this kind of therapeutic exercise to gentle music, of the kind you might have in a yoga class or at a massage, it makes it feel like luxurious self-care.

Accountability

Having someone to check in with can make all the difference. Completing the programme with a friend or family member can be very helpful. Or have someone to check in with every time you complete a day.

Accountability doesn't even need to be a "person". It could mean posting on social media, or keeping a journal. A basic check in outside of yourself can make all the difference.

Email check in

I have put together an email support series especially for this programme. If you sign up you will receive regular emails to help you stay on track for the full 12 weeks. Sign up here:
https://www.subscribepage.com/h0p3t1_copy

Rest

Rest is important for 2 main reasons, and those are even more important to people with chronic fatigue issues and connective tissue disorders.
1) Your body needs to repair.
Exercise causes tiny amounts of damage in all your tissues, it needs to, it's part of the "use it or lose it" process that stimulates the tissues to become stronger, without that stimulus, your muscle and bone is considered surplus to requirements and slowly broken down.
It is vitally important that your tissues are given the optimal opportunity to repair and grow. Which is why your programme starts slow, spacing out those strength workouts, and why I strongly encourage a well considered rest protocol.

2) Your nervous system needs to reset. Your autonomic nervous system has 2 modes, "fight or flight" and "rest and digest". Work stress, exercise, even watching action movies, puts your system on high alert, which is fine and healthy. But it is important that your body returns to its resting state afterwards. People with chronic pain are often in their alert state for large

amounts of time, and this state can aggravate or even trigger co-morbid conditions like fibromyalgia

It's important that you move on your rest days, a gentle walk is ideal.

Make sure you are getting enough sleep, set yourself up with a bedtime that allows you around 7 ½ hours sleep and see if it feels like you need more or less from there.

Daily downtime to reset your nervous system is a great recovery habit to get into - colouring, meditation, lying down and listening to music, any kind of deliberate relaxation to help put your brain into rest mode. I worked with an occupational therapist to organise the pacing of my day. I find that planning a 10-15 minute break before and after my most demanding activities really helpful.

Failing that, consider alternating your physical and mental tasks so that you can break up the stressors on your systems.

If you feel sore or stiff as a result of exercising (which is totally normal when you change up your routine), have a long soak in a warm bath with a cup of epsom salts added.

If you want to develop better habits around a healthy lifestyle, I would thoroughly recommend my book "Break the Diet Habit", which delivers a programme for a healthy approach to mindset, lifestyle and nutrition.

Nutrition

You need to fuel your training and recovery properly. While this is not the place for an extended nutrition primer, I'm going to drop the following hints:

Protein - try to eat a portion of lean protein with every meal (3 meals a day). You need it for recovery. A portion of a protein rich food, like egg white or lean meat, is about the size and thickness of your palm. You will need 1-2 portions per meal.

Lean protein means things like chicken breast or lean beef, low fat Greek yoghurt or skyr. If you eat a plant based diet, look for high protein carbohydrates like beans and quinoa.

Vegetables - eat a portion of colourful veg, or 2, with every meal. A portion of vegetables is a big handful. Colourful vegetables are full of micronutrients, and mixing them up means you get a broader variety of vitamins and minerals. I don't promote the use of supplements except for Vitamin D (which is really important for people with EDS as we tend to have lower levels), but if you have issues with fatigue you might like to consider a B complex, Manganese and Magnesium, have a chat to your healthcare provider about it - I take a sports multivitamin with all these in, with an awareness that not all the ingredients are useful, but it's not harmful either.

Carbohydrates - most people don't need reminding of this as generally we all love carbs, but now is not the time to start cutting them. While it is fashionable lately to suggest carbs are the root of all evil, minimally processed, wholegrain carbohydrates are easily accessible fuel for your body.

Some people feel great on low carbohydrate diets, some will feel very tired and sluggish, I would suggest your starting point should align with the most evidence-based advice, which is to eat a portion of carbs with each meal.

A portion of a carb rich food (like rice, potato, pasta etc) is about the same size as your fist.

Fats - Healthy fats, like nuts, avocado, vegetable oils and rich dairy are important for your health. A portion of healthy fat is about the size of your thumb, so maybe ¼ avocado, 10 almonds or a tablespoon of olive oil.

Water - stay hydrated, drink a big glass of water with every meal, after training, and sip from a bottle during training. If you aren't used to exercise you may find you're dehydrating.

Equipment

I've kept the equipment out of this programme, saving some things you might find about the house - like chairs - a foam roller and a stretchy band.

Bands are very cheap to buy and come in a variety of strengths, I would recommend a set of light, medium and heavy so you can add some progression if it gets too easy. Some bands are made of latex and you may wish to avoid those if there is a risk of allergy.

Foam rollers are also quite easy to find cheaply online, I'd recommend a smooth one to begin with. You may find some areas are hard to roll while you are still building core strength, so you will also need a tennis ball or massage ball to substitute.

I've included a couple of exercises that need light dumbbells, feel free to substitute a tin of soup/beans.

Flares and Injury

Our goal is to reduce your instances of flare ups and injuries by improving your strength and co-ordination in order to stabilise your joints and improve your movement patterns.

But living with HSD means that you are likely to still experience flares and injuries from time to time, and it is necessary to address that.

If you are having a period where you are feeling more tired or in more generalised pain than usual, this is a good time to consider using a deload week to reduce the demand on your body.

Skipping exercise entirely carries the risk of regression and losing the progress you have made, but a deload week can often help progress when you are "hitting a wall".

If you are considering dropping a workout because you feel bad, consider "will this workout make me feel better or worse?". Sometimes if we feel sluggish, exercise really helps. But if you honestly feel like it won't, then take a stroll (if you can), rest up, and try again tomorrow.

Acute injuries like sprains are common in unstable joints. I've tried to avoid exercises that are at all risky, but then, we can dislocate things in our sleep, so we best be prepared!

If you acquire a new injury, RICE (Rest, Ice Compress, Elevate).

Avoid putting too much strain on the area until it feels better, but use it gently if you can. Seek medical attention if you feel it's not resolving. If an older injury continues to feel weak or painful, speak to a physiotherapist about rehab.

Wherever possible, try to keep exercising around your injury. Do as much as you can with your non-affected areas. Consider water based exercise to avoid loading joints.

While people with HSD often progress slowly in fitness, we also tend to lose it quickly. The downward spiral of injury, ceasing exercise and becoming weaker (so more prone to more injuries) is very real and should be avoided.

Your programme

This is what your week looks like:

Cardio

Your cardio exercise is going to consist of a "brisk" walk. But this is your version of "brisk", so move at a pace that feels a little challenging.

You can gauge how hard you are working by noticing your breathing, you should be breathing harder than normal, but still able to talk. You could hold a conversation, but might need some big breaths or breaks between sentences.

You are also welcome to substitute this for swimming, cycling, dancing, whatever keeps you at the right level of exertion, but just make sure you maintain your effort for the full duration stated in your programme.

I also heartily encourage low level activity for whatever duration you feel able. The recommendation is that you are active for at least 30 minutes, 5 days a week, and you can even break that down into 3 bouts.

So let's say it's cardio day in week 1, you could do a 10 minute brisk walk, then continue at a relaxed pace for a further 20 minutes. Or you could do your 10 minute walk, then 10 minutes of housework and a final 10 minutes pottering in the garden later on.

However, please remember we are aiming for slow, steady progress, so it's reasonable to build up to this if it feels like a big leap from where you're at right now.

Mobility

This is where you will work on freeing up tight areas and developing a healthy range of motion. We will be using three different methods here:

Self myofascial release

Think of Self myofascial release as home-massage. The aim is to encourage the nervous system to let go of overactive muscle and encourage free movement. You will apply pressure to the muscle, seeking out tender "trigger points" then maintain the pressure for around 30 seconds until you feel the tender, knotty area melt away. You can use a foam roller or a ball to do this. Some people like to use a massage gun, and while I wouldn't suggest you rush out and buy one, if you have one, you can use it.

Check out the videos linked in Part 4 of this book for more detailed instruction.

Dynamic stretching

Gently moving and "feeling out" your range of motion warms up the joints and stabilising muscles whilst also being a safe way to improve healthy range of motion. You'll find these in the warm up.

Static stretching

These are optional and are found in the latter part of the mobility session. You may find these helpful and use them every time, you may wish to use them only one session a week, or you may omit them completely. They are there to reinforce the work you've done in the self myofascial release and you will likely benefit if you are finding trigger points in the associated muscle.

Resistance training

This bit is about building some strength in your muscles. More precisely, this programme contains the stabilisation phase (after which we would move into a muscular endurance phase)

We will be working on strengthening isolated muscles, as well as performing some movements that involve groups of muscles working together, and some balancing

Your exercise library

To keep your programme nice and clear, I have put descriptions and video links to all the exercises in Part 4 of this book.

The 12 week plan

I've broken your programme down into 3, 4 week blocks. Consistency and repetition are important, so the structure of each week within a month is the same, but we change things up as we progress from month to month.

If you reach the end of a month and feel like you're not ready to move on, don't feel pressured to. There is no reason not to repeat another week or more if you wish to.

I have also included a deload (rest) week. Ideally this goes inbetween week 8 and 9, but you can use this if you have a week where you feel more tired than usual, premenstrual, or have stuff going on in your life that means you don't have so much energy to devote to fitness.

Your workout

Go through the warm up at the start of every session, and the cool down at the end.

If you are doing mobility, then cardio straight after, you can warm up before mobility and cool down after cardio. If you split the session you will need to warm up before each activity. There is no need to cool down after mobility if that is all you do.

Sets are the number of rounds of each exercise, reps are the number of repetitions, rest is the break you take between rounds. So if your sets/reps/rest is 2/10/30s, you are going to do 10 repetitions of the exercise, rest for 30 seconds, then do another 10 before moving onto the next exercise.

Tempo refers to the timing of the exercise. 2/2 means you take 2 seconds on each phase (there and back again) of the movement. 4-2-1 means you take 4 seconds to lower under tension, 2 seconds hold at the end of the movement, and one second to push/pull back against gravity. The video demonstrations for each exercise explain this in more detail.

EXERCISE WITH EDS

12 WEEK PRIMER

	SESSION 1	SESSION 2	SESSION 3
WEEK 1-4	MOBILITY 1 CARDIO – 10 MINUTES	STABILITY 1 CARDIO – 10 MINUTES	MOBILITY 1 CARDIO – 10 MINUTES
WEEK 5-8	STABILITY 1 CARDIO – 15 MINUTES	MOBILITY 1 CARDIO – 15 MINUTES	STABILITY 1 CARDIO – 15 MINUTES
DELOAD	MOBILITY 1 CARDIO – 10 MINUTES	MOBILITY 1	MOBILITY 1 CARDIO – 10 MINUTES
WEEK 9-12	STABILITY 2 CARDIO – 20 MINUTES	MOBILITY 1 CARDIO – 30 MINUTES	STABILITY 2 CARDIO – 20 MINUTES

WARM UP & COOL DOWN

EXERCISE	DURATION
March on spot	60s
Jog on spot (or march faster)	60s
Standing spinal twist	20s
Elbow circles	20s
Jog on spot (or march faster)	60s
Step back with overhead reach	30s
Alternate toe touch	30s

MOBILITY 1

WARM UP FIRST

FOAM ROLLER OR MASSAGE BALL	DURATION
Gastrocnemius (calf)	60s
TFL/IT band	60s
Latissiumus Dorsi	60s
OPTIONAL	
Chest/pecs stretch	30s
Lat ball stretch	30s
Lying hip flexor stretch	30s
Gastrocnemius (calf) stretch	30s

STABILITY 1

WARM UP FIRST, COOL DOWN AFTERWARDS

SETS/REPS/REST	EXERCISE	TEMPO
2/20/20s	Dead bug	2-2
2/15/20s	Lying pelvic tuck	4-2-1
2/3 each side	Single leg balance	10 second hold
2/15/30s	Wall push up	4-2-1
2/15/30s	Band pull apart	4-2-1
2/15/30s	Lateral shoulder raise	4-2-1
2/12/30s	Chair squat	4-2-1

STABILITY 2
WARM UP FIRST, COOL DOWN AFTERWARDS

SETS/REPS/REST	EXERCISE	TEMPO
2/16/20s	Straight leg dead bug	2-2
2/12/20s	Glute bridge	4-2-1
2/3 each side	Single leg balance with reach	2-2
2/12/30s	Bench push up	4-2-1
2/12/30s	Band row	4-2-1
2/12/30s	Single leg scaption	4-2-1
2/12/30s	Step up to balance	4-2-1

I've kept this programme as simple and concise as possible, because I want it to be easy to follow and easy to motivate yourself to complete.

Full videos of each session are available (links in Part 4) so that you can follow along if you find that helpful or motivating.

The next step

On completion of the 12 weeks you are likely to find yourself in one of 3 places:

Ready to enter mainstream exercise

You feel like you can push your cardio harder and you're not so out of breath. Your joints are feeling a bit stronger and you might be experiencing less "wobbles" or pain.

Great news. Look around for an entry level class, talk to an in-house trainer at the gym and ask for a basic programme, give something new a go!

Stay safe by explaining your situation to your instructors, don't force yourself to do something that hurts, or has hurt you in the past, ask for an alternative. Remember that you still need to take your progress slowly, maybe try one class a week to start with, and keep up your mobility and cardio from the last block of the programme.

In need of a little more support

You may feel like you want to stay in the last block of the programme for a couple more weeks, or find something of a similar, or mildly progressed level.

If you would like more of this kind of programme, created with your needs in mind, I offer a programming service as part of my online personal training.

Committed to a focused plan

It may be that your unique body has some issues that a general programme is only skimming. Perhaps you have a strong movement dysfunction or a particular area that is causing strife. It may be that improving on a general level highlights an area of weakness.

In this case you could benefit from an individualised corrective exercise programme. This is something I offer as an online service, or with in-person assessment and coaching for those within range. Alternatively another Corrective Exercise Specialist or Sports physiotherapist may be able to help you.

Part 3 - Going deeper

In this section I am including some longer pieces of writing about questions I have been asked before. They are edited versions of articles published on my blog at blog.firelotusfitness.com

Training clients with Ehlers Danlos Syndrome - a primer for Fitpros

I wrote this piece for fitness professionals, I am including it here, because you may wish to pass it on.

...

When you have a rare health condition, it's pretty exciting when you encounter someone who knows about it. Even more so when you encounter people who are interested in it and more importantly, understanding how to bridge the gap and work with it.

This is why I am really happy to be seeing more and more fitness professionals asking "I have a client with Ehlers Danlos Syndrome, what do I need to know?"

Quick disclaimer before we start - I'm not a medic, and this is not for medics. Please seek specific medical input from your/your client's health care professionals. And with that we get to our first point.

Scope of practice.

Quick, check your job title. Are you a personal trainer or coach? Good, because that's who I am aiming this at. More importantly I am assuming you are not a rheumatologist, or geneticist - so it is not your place to diagnose. You are not a physiotherapist, so it is not your place to treat or rehabilitate injuries. You aren't a dietitian, so you are not going to prescribe supplements or offer therapeutic meal plans.

If those things are needed always refer.

You might be a corrective exercise specialist - this is brilliant, because you have the skillset to work at reducing postural issues and movement dysfunctions which are really common in people with EDS and contribute to a lot of their pain and injuries.

If you are a personal trainer you are able to help your client overcome barriers to exercise and train safely through a progressive programme. Good stuff.

So with that out of the way...

What even is Ehlers Danlos Syndrome?

EDS is one of a number of genetic connective tissue disorders which are often referred to as Hypermobility disorders as the most obvious symptom is hypermobile joints.

So let's break this down - Genetic means that it is caused by a glitch in the DNA code that is essentially our body's recipe for collagen. It is usually inherited from our parents, but spontaneous mutations can also cause it. There are genetic tests for some, but not all types of EDS.

While we often talk about EDS in terms of the effects on the human movement system, it is important to be aware that collagen is an important structural component in all the body systems, and the effects of producing collagen that is effectively too elastic has a broad and diverse range of effects.

There are also several types of EDS, and some people, like me, have symptoms that cross types.

For more info check this out.
https://www.ehlers-danlos.org/what-is-eds/

How does this affect me as a trainer?

As a fitpro you don't need to know everything about EDS, so here's the run down on the stuff you should be aware of...

Hypermobility

Actually I feel like this term is a misnomer from a fitness perspective (but not a medical one as we speak slightly different languages). People with EDS have a larger than usual range of motion in their joints (not necessarily all their joints). But they are flexible not mobile, that is to say the range of strong controlled motion might even be less, but the passive range of motion can be dangerously unstable.

Hypermobility alone isn't an issue. A person who is hypermobile but has no other symptoms would be just fine. Much attention is paid to this, most obvious symptom, when in truth, flexibility is not a detrimental trait, but you know what is?

Poor proprioception

People with EDS don't have a good idea of where their body is in space. Most people have good feedback mechanisms that let them know when they are reaching the limit of their range of motion, so they often have highly dysfunctional movement patterns.

Look for hyperextended knees when standing, hyperextended elbows in plank, fingers flat to the floor in burpees when the palms are still off the floor, excessive wrist flexion when benching. Correcting these can simply be an issue of bringing awareness and training a new "normal" into the client's muscle memory.

Failing to correct these will lead to a greatly increased risk of injury - sprains and dislocations are very common in EDS, you can't afford to let poor form slide.

Postural and movement dysfunctions

Due to a lack of strength in the ligaments, holding good posture can be an issue with EDS. Hyperlordosis due to lumbar weakness can throw out the lumbo pelvic hip complex putting the back and knees at risk.

Equally excessive pronation can lead to knee issues and affect the LPHC. Many EDSers have flat feet, or feet that move in and out of pronation. Watch the client in movement as well as at rest as some areas will "drop in and out" of their issues.

And you'll see all kinds of variations between individuals, our bodies are special and unpredictable.

Fatigue

Chronic fatigue is a common symptom in people with EDS. There's many reasons for this and it is worth addressing a few separately.

Sleep can be an issue because of pain or difficulty in getting comfortable. I personally have subluxed shoulders and hips from sleeping awkwardly. Several of the conditions which are linked with EDS, like fibromyalgia and anxiety also cause sleep issues.

Moving around with EDS is also just that bit more tiring, the effort it takes to move well while feeling out your movements with poor proprioception and the extra muscle effort it takes to stabilise the joints means that they are working that bit harder to achieve the same ends.

Consider this in your programming, particularly in the early stages and understanding that endurance will be initially lower than expected.

Pain, which can be generalised and chronic, or specific to an injury, is simply draining. Living with chronic pain means filtering out a persistent "background noise" and it's just wearing. Many standard analgesics don't work on chronic pain, and one of the symptoms of EDS can be a reduced efficacy of certain drug types.

Kinesiophobia

People with unstable joints injure easily. I have sprained ankles walking down the street, broken a foot by rolling my ankle getting off the sofa (I didn't notice until I heard the crack), dislocated kneecaps for no obvious reason and popped ribs by sneezing.

This along with chronic pain can make people with EDS reluctant to exercise. Which isn't helped when the advice many people give us on exercise is "don't" or "go careful".

Building up activity slowly focusing at first on alignment and just getting moving is a good start. I get people walking on the flat first. Aim for small victories and consistent progress.

Whatever happens, be aware that a reluctance to move (which can even play out as a physical inability to do so) is a symptom of the condition, not necessarily a lack of motivation.

Dysautonomia

The autonomic nervous system regulates all our unconscious functions, everything from heart rate to digestive transit and hormone release. For some of us, it's wrong. It's just wrong.

PoTS is really common as is PoBS (the opposite, where your heart doesn't adjust to a change in posture or activity correctly). Blood pressure regulation is confused by stretchy blood vessels.

What you need to know is that your EDS client may not react physiologically as you expect. Be aware of this in high intensity exercise and you may need to consider sequencing your workout so as to avoid getting up and down off the floor repeatedly for instance.

Digestive issues and nutrition

If you are a nutritionist (or perhaps if you aren't) you need to be aware that EDS also has a role to play in messing around with the guts. IBS is really common, as are general issues with digestive transit. The guts are just too stretchy.

Sudden changes in diet, exposure to intolerances, a change in fibre content or water intake could all throw a spanner in the works. In essence I am advocating good coaching protocols, make changes small, achievable and slow, take feedback, adjust accordingly.

People with EDS often have vitamin D deficiency and it works out quite well that (in the UK) Vit D is the only one fitpros are supposed to recommend as a supplement within scope of practice, so go ahead and do that if you like.

A healthy balanced diet is always your go to. Gear towards recovery, that's super important. Some people talk about collagen supplementation, some people say that's daft because the client is making faulty collagen and feeding them good collagen will never change that. However, feeding to recover and build connective tissue strength is going to help them to produce the best result *for them*.

Other issues to note

Costochondritis, inflammation around the sternum is an extremely painful condition that can be mistaken for a heart attack. All chest pain should be taken seriously and investigated.

Bruising and skin damage. Due to delicate capillaries and fragile skin, clients with EDS are more susceptible to minor skin injuries. Also they can have super stretchy skin which is going to mess your skinfold tests right up.

What can and can't an EDS athlete do?

Now here is a minefield... Let's mythbust....

Hypermobile people shouldn't stretch

To say this is to assume that each person is universally and symmetrically flexible in all joints. Remember what I said about postural and movement dysfunction? It is very usual for certain muscles to tighten up as part of a complex misalignment. That hyperlordosis means short hip flexors. You can't correct it without releasing the tight areas. Injuries and compensations due to injury can also cause decreased mobility or imbalance.

Progressive stretching on already hyperflexible joints is not a good plan. Corrective stretching and mobility work are still valid.

Hypermobile people shouldn't do yoga

I've written a separate piece on this, which appears later in this book.

Hypermobile people shouldn't run.

High impact, repetitive movements can set you up for joint injuries. However there are many runners with EDS and if that is how they choose to be active, we can support them in that. Issues to focus on would include a good gait with midfoot landing, and a parallel programme of strength training to focus on stability in the ankle, knee and hip.

Hypermobile people can't do CrossFit

The issue with CrossFit here, or any sport that requires and athlete to perform high intensity, high impact movement under extreme fatigue, is that the risk of injury is high. Anyone pushing themselves like this will get sloppy with form and that's just a bit more likely if that person already has proprioception issues, fatigue and joint instability.

Is it still possible for someone with EDS to enjoy CrossFit if they are appropriately fit? Absolutely. The question is one of readiness. Is it the best option? Probably not, but if that's what motivates them to keep fit, more power to them.

Hypermobile people shouldn't lift heavy.

Well I do. And I'm not alone. Strength training has been the single most effective way for me to manage my joint instability. I get less injuries, less falls and less pain as a result.

With any kind of training/activity, the trick is to approach it intelligently, not to discount it from the outset.

Top Tips for Training bendy zebras

So with all that in mind, let's summarise....

1. Listen to your client, properly. If they say they can't do something, believe them, and then find out why. Ask questions, look at the big picture. And help them through it.

2. Start slow, like super slow, don't push them and see what it takes to break them, better to start by instilling movement habits and good form.

3. Alignment and form always. Train good movement habits, correct dysfunction. Make sure that is all in place before attempting anything further.

4. Expect slow progress. Also unusual progress. I can build muscle fast, but developing the corresponding connective tissue strength takes much longer.

5. Expect rapid decline. Time off is a killer, be prepared to take some steps back after a break.

6. Think recovery. Think sleep, think stress management, think nutrition.

7. Don't be afraid to rest and deload, but avoid stopping completely.

8. Remember your client is an individual. Fitting into the EDS box for diagnosis doesn't mean that every EDS client will be the same.

9. Programme intelligently. Look for value in movements. Look at kinetic chains, co-ordination, balance. Consider managing fatigue. This is not the place for beasting or heroics.

10. If in doubt, refer out.

In conclusion

I have encountered many people with EDS who have complained that they cannot find a personal trainer who will work with them due to doubts about their health. Those people are often afraid to exercise without guidance and end up inactive and deteriorating. As a profession we can do better than that.

A trainer who is willing to listen and learn more about their clients is worth their weight in gold. Be one of those.

Yoga and hypermobility

I wanted to properly address a question that keeps coming up on various hypermobility and EDS forums that I frequent.

It always goes like this. Someone asks a question like "I've just been diagnosed with hypermobility, I've been told I can't do yoga anymore..."

The responses are always a mixture of "yes, my doctor/physio told me yoga was the worst thing I could do for my hypermobility" and "I do yoga and it's been the best thing for my hypermobility".

So what gives?

Well, I'm firmly in the "yoga is useful" camp, and I have to disclose that. I'm a yoga practitioner of around 20 years and a perinatal yoga teacher, as well as a personal trainer and bendy person.

While I have the deepest respect for the medical professionals who are giving out this advice, their expertise doesn't usually extend into yoga, and I think often these comments are coming from a misunderstanding of what yoga is about, how it works and what actually happens to a hypermobile body while training yoga. I'd never suggest that anyone went against the advice of their medical carers, but it is an opportunity to open up a conversation and find out exactly what they are objecting to, and why.

So let's break it down.

There are different kinds of yoga.

Loads. Millions. Many of them are related to each other, in that students of a particular teacher went off and started their own schools which have subtle differences, but some of them are wildly different.

Yoga has been heavily appropriated by the Western world, and in some cases, what originated as a spiritual lifestyle of mind-body connection, has turned into an instagrammable pursuit of "perfect" aesthetics and visually impressive feats. Or it has been modified to fit Western fitness ideals of physical challenge, sweatiness and feats of strength. If that's your bag, then that's absolutely fine - we should all be doing the exercise we love most.

But I've also encountered hypermobile people who have been to one of these "high performance" yoga classes and found it wholly unsuitable. This shouldn't be a reason to write off yoga completely. It just means that teacher or style wasn't right for that person at that time.

The confusion about what yoga is

The primary reason our zebras are being told to stay clear of yoga is "yoga makes you more flexible, you are already too flexible"

This is a classic misunderstanding of the purpose and practice of yoga. Yoga is about building healthy function and movement patterns into the body, in a mindful way. It's about tuning into what your body is capable of, and what your body needs, right now, without judgement. This is what is lost in the Western picture perfect asana culture. It's not about "achieving" the asana, it's about the journey of figuring out where the imbalance of strength, mobility and alignment is in your body, about acknowledging it and caring for it.

Yoga is also about a lot more than asana. It's about breathing, which improves core strength, cardiovascular and autonomic function (all important for zebras). It's about being aware of your body, its position, alignment and the changes within it (also super important....) and it's about meditation and relaxation to reduce stressors in the body (the sort of thing that can trigger fatigue, pain and comorbid conditions like fibromyalgia).

Again, if you go to a class and the sole focus is forcing yourself into a human pretzel shape - you are missing out on some of the best bits of yoga, and that's not what I'm talking about when I say yoga is great for hypermobility syndrome.

Yoga for alignment and good movement patterns

Many of the yoga sequences and poses are designed to promote good biomechanics. We practice the movements slowly and mindfully, until they are set into our muscle memory and start creeping out in our everyday movements. The posture, the gait, the process of moving the body, with awareness, balance and core strength, applying the right muscles in the right order with the right balance. It's exactly what people with poor proprioception and unstable joints need.

I've spoken to people who were advised "if you do yoga you must be careful not to extend beyond a healthy range of movement". Well, yes. That is exactly what you will be working on! One of the big problems with being hypermobile, is that we don't have a clear "feeling" of a safe range of motion, by the time a joint reaches the limit of its movement, it has already gone into a position which is potentially unsafe. We do this all the time, when walking, standing, sitting... in our sleep. Yoga practice gives us a window of time to focus purely on getting that right.

Being hypermobile doesn't necessarily mean being bendy everywhere

The most common diagnostic procedure for hypermobility is the Beighton score. It is a measure of how generalised your joint hypermobility is. It's not always accurate because it only covers 9 joints out of dozens that could be affected, it's also not indicative of severity. I know people with

EDS who have a score of 4/9 and have severe movement impairment. I have a score of 8/9 and with management I pass as healthy.

When I encounter hypermobile PT clients, I am always fascinated by how their unique bodies come together. The hypermobility is not always bilateral (I have one hypermobile wrist and one "normal" one). Often they will have a large range of motion in an internal hip rotation, but very limited external rotation. Often years of "interesting" posture (standing or sitting) have caused some really unusual chain reactions between joint sites. I used to have one pronated foot and one supernated! Hip instability goes unnoticed and manifests in the knees.

When working on postural correction through strength/fitness training, we think on two sides of the coin, what needs to be stronger, and what is too tight?

So what I am getting at is that even someone with hypermobility will have areas that need to be stretched or otherwise released. Probably moreso than the average person.

One of the cool things about yoga, is that you find those areas in the process of working through the movements, and as you work on those movements, getting deeper into the asana, the right parts are gradually released.

Flexibility vs mobility - the language barrier

Here's a fun factoid. The medical definition of mobility is "the ability of a joint to be moved through its range in different planes."

Notice that describes a passive process. Like the Beighton test, it is about how far the joint can be moved, by an external force.

In fitness we call that flexibility.

In fitness terms, mobility is an active process. Mobility is the ability to move a joint using the appropriate musculature. So for instance doing a floor split, using gravity, could be described as flexibility.

But doing a standing split, in yoga or dance, would be mobility, as you have to use your muscles to raise and hold the leg.

So when I say that yoga (or pilates or suchlike) increases mobility, I am saying that it increases the range of motion through which the joint has strength and stability. What a medical professional hears though, is that it makes the joint less stable by increasing passive range of motion.

Two very different things. The first being something many hypermobile people lack, and need to improve their symptoms, the second being a recipe for dislocations.

So what we have come back to, is the need for communication. Clear dialogue and understanding.

I regularly come across people with hypermobility who have been told they need to retire from their favourite sport, or that no one with their condition should consider yoga, or strength training above very low resistance levels, or running. Yet I have also met numerous hypermobile yogis, powerlifters, crossfitters and marathon runners!

Exercise is good for our bodies. It increases connective tissue strength and develops musculature to support our joints. The top experts in rehab for hypermobility recognise that exercise you enjoy and want to take part in is ultimately more effective than conventional "rehab" if only because you actually do it!

So ask questions, seek second opinions, work with all the right experts to figure out your balance between what you enjoy, what works in your body and what makes you feel at your best.

Training through chronic illness - living life on the edge.

I'm living a double life.

My superhero persona goes to the gym and lifts enormous weights. She's vital and has her life together. Endless to-do lists in a bullet journal, juggling work and kids and being an athlete and performer with theatrical effortlessness.

Then there's the secret side people don't see, where I lie on the sofa in my flare day leggings and fleece, clutching a cup of tea for the slight relief the warmth affords my stiff, clawed hands.

I know I'm not the only one. I know a lot of athletes living with chronic illness. Outwardly fitter and busier than the average person, inwardly wracked with pain and fatigue.

There are two ways people tend to interpret this. Either we are not as sick as we claim, or we are stupidly putting our health at risk doing sport that seems counter-intuitive to our well being. The reality is a lot more complicated. I wanted to formulate a decent answer to "why do you do this to yourself", so here goes....

Training as therapy

I have Ehlers Danlos Syndrome and Fibromyalgia. Both are conditions that cause chronic pain and fatigue, but both also have "exercise" recommended as part of the management plan. There is a fair bit of discussion about how that should actually happen.

The basic recommendations are walking and strength training (to stabilise joints). And that is exactly where I start when I am working with personal training clients with hypermobility or similar chronic issues.

But everyone needs a why, and I can honestly say that things like "not falling over so much" just don't stand the test of time when you are doing theraband exercises 5 times a day. If we are going to be consistent with our training, we need...

- a programme we enjoy
- goals that feel valuable, with frequent reward
- a sense of progress
- habits we can build into our lives
- grit and determination.

So my bodyweight and theraband exercises became freeweight exercises, and freeweights became powerlifting Walking became running. Not overnight, but over several years of gradual, careful, patient progress.

I started to understand what I could be capable of (and what I clearly wasn't capable of...) I have far fewer subluxations and dislocations, because I am stronger. It works.

The side effects of training

Training makes me feel good. The post exercise endorphins mute my screaming central nervous system, if only briefly.

The achievements and little wins, getting to feel like a competent badass. They keep me showing up week after week. For me it's worth the work.

Even the post exercise muscle soreness feels good because I worked for it. It turns pain from "what did I do to deserve this" to "I did a great job today".

The price of management

Of course it's not that simple. Exercising takes energy (or spoons), Energy that I might want for stuff like, cooking dinner, doing a grocery shop, going to work and earning a living, that sort of thing. I have to decide what I am going to prioritise. Then ultimately, the benefit of exercise, is that it keeps me well enough to do more exercise.

When I started, training took more out of me than I got back, but over time it has levelled out and my increased fitness and vitality pays off, but I still feel it's mostly a "spoons neutral" process.

I could live at my desk, use splints and walking aids when I need to move and ultimately have no more or less "spare" energy (but a lower turnover). I've been there. It's OK, I understand and respect anyone's right to do that. Having boisterous children and loving stuff like dance and being active outdoors makes it worthwhile for me to invest in the ability to be more active.

I like feeling good in my body. I love my physical capability. I am prepared to make sacrifices for it. Also I can eat a lot more cake this way.

Pacing and recovery

Some of the powerlifters I speak to are lifting 5-6 times a week. I don't. I train 4 days a week with great programming from a coach who understands that progress isn't about training until you drop as much as possible.

On top of that I teach 2 fitness classes and one dance class a week and do a short cardio session if I feel it's a good call. In between I rest. I manage my day around making sure I keep mobile, but low key, sleep well, eat well and give myself the best opportunity to grow strong ready for the next session.

Managing my own work schedule makes an enormous difference for me. I can deliberately put pacing breaks in my day to let my nervous system wind down. Managing my tasks in an organised fashion means I get less stress from late deadlines and panic over forgotten responsibilities. Low stress hormones means better recovery and less for my systems to have to handle.

With this in mind I have also got really good at boundaries. I used to do everything for everyone because well, I'm a helpful kind of person. Now I have to think carefully, I am literally donating my life force and I am very careful about where that goes!

The relentless habit

A sad truth about EDS, is that gains are slow and losses are rapid. It takes a long time to build connective tissue strength because my connective tissue is always going to be lacking. But also, if I stop training, I lose strength very quickly. I am well aware that I am potentially a few weeks "off" away from being back with serious mobility problems.

It's also very easy to decide not to train because of injury. I adjust my programme as necessary to rest injuries without compromising progress.

I subluxed a kneecap a couple of months back and it's been tricky since. I've asked my coach to drop all lunges out of my programme. I can still squat, it's just the unilateral loading that is problematic, so there's still squats and leg press in my routine, building much needed stability around the joint.

Being a health bore

If I went back in time a few years and told my past self what my nutrition and rest regimen looks like now, she would laugh at me and say "no way". But over time I have been figuring out what feels best in my body and I have started to realise that some things just aren't worth it.

I gave up wearing non-practical shoes, because I wanted to be well for dance. Now I've come for other lifestyle factors.

A couple of months ago, I stopped drinking alcohol completely. I've not been a "drinker" for a long time, but I realised that even the odd glass of wine was wiping me out the next day, and it's just not worth feeling that awful for.

I go to bed by 10.30pm, every night. I am boringly stringent about this. I can't function the next day otherwise.

I haven't "cut" anything from my diet, but I do make note of the foods that make me feel well and the foods that don't. I need enough protein and vegetables. I have to drink plenty of water. Stodgy, refined carbs don't sit well with me and too much of them make me feel gross. I accept this and act on it, the result is eating a healthy and minimally processed diet. I'm not strict with myself, but most of the time I recognise that going "off plan" is going to make me feel ill, or compromise my ability to train, which is important to me.

Sacrifice and balance

Dropping some things has been easy, others less so. Recognising that I can't spread myself too thin means harshly pruning back on many aspects of my life. Being well for my clients and family comes first. Anyone else wanting my time or energy has to take a ticket and might have a long wait.

I have had to make ruthless and sometimes painful decisions that prioritise what is essential and most important to me.

I once told my occupational therapist - I walk a fine tightrope in order to be this functional. I can't afford to take on extra load, look around at the scenery or stray off the path.

But it's my path, and I love it and it's totally worth it.

Part 4 - Exercise library

Warm up

Standing spinal twist - Standing with your feet apart and arms relaxed, twist the torso looking back over one shoulder, then change direction.
Elbow circles - Touching your shoulder, circle the elbows, slowly in as large a range of motion as you can. Make sure you circle in both directions.
Alternate toe touch - From standing, feet wide, reach the right hand down towards the left foot, keeping the back flat, stand up straight again, reach the left hand to the right foot.
Step back with overhead reach - From standing, take a short step back with the right foot, reach both arms up to above the head, slightly on the left side, step back to start. Repeat on the other side.

A full video of your warm up is here:
https://youtu.be/Ced_w6WfYY8

Mobility 1

Foam rolling

Gastrocnemius (calf) - Sit on the floor with your legs straight in front of you. Keeping your back straight, slowly roll from just below the knee, to just before the achilles tendon. Pause and hold on any tender areas.
There are 2 options on the videos, try both and see which feels more productive for you.
https://youtu.be/KaPsujtbYFs
https://youtu.be/qmfRaeCBdBk

TFL/IT band - Lying on your side, roll from just below the greater trochanter (the bony bit on your hip) to just above the knee. If you cannot support yourself in this position, take a tennis ball, or massage ball, and apply gentle rolling pressure along this area.
https://youtu.be/3iz1or5QKY4
Lattissimus dorsi - Lying on your side, place your underneath arm palm up and pointing away from your feet. Roll from just below the armpit to mid back (bra strap area). If you cannot support yourself in this position, use the stretch below instead.
https://youtu.be/3EP4qouqdO0

Static stretching

Chest (pec) - sit or stand tall with your arms out to the side and your elbows bent at a right angle (like a fork with a pea in the middle). squeeze your shoulder blades together and ease your elbows back.
https://youtu.be/7wnwLQ7CuRQ
Gastrocnemius (calf) - Stand in front of a wall with one foot in front of the other. Lean into the wall keeping your back heel on the floor until you feel a comfortable tension.
https://youtu.be/27Vkhx6kVr8
Lying hip flexor - lying with your bottom on the edge of a firm surface, allow one leg to hang while drawing the opposite knee into the chest.
https://youtu.be/1R9Gj2NNnXU
Lattissimus dorsi - place yourself on all 4s in front of a low table, chair or fitness ball. Raise one arm into line with your ear (parallel to the floor) and rest it, thumb up, on the surface in front of you.
https://youtu.be/9xYCnTAnM7U

Stability 1

Dead bug - Lie on your back with your knees bent, thighs at a right angle to the floor and calves parallel to the floor. Raise your arms at a right angle to the floor. Now drop the right leg, to tap the floor, while also dropping the left arm back above your head. Return to the start and switch sides.
https://youtu.be/rPLCbrK25d8

Lying pelvic tuck -lie on your back with your knees bent and feet on the floor, be aware of the hollow (mouse hole) under the low back. Tuck your tailbone and use your low abs to flatten your lower back into the floor, squashing the mouse hold for 2s and slowly release (4s)
https://youtu.be/hb5d_E26E2s
Single leg balance - stand tall in good posture, lift one foot slightly off the floor. Use the back of a chair for more support if needed.
https://youtu.be/PxcJduiHv4o
Wall push up - stand in front of a wall, at arm's length. Place your hands on the wall, slightly wide of your shoulders. Bend your elbows, keeping them close to your sides to lean into the wall (4s), hold for 2 seconds, then push away under control.
https://youtu.be/meYsyITvVnk
Band pull apart - Stand or sit upright, arms front of you palms up. Grip the resistance band in your hands and extend the shoulders, moving the arm through 90 degrees. You should feel this in-between your shoulder blades. Hold with the arms extended for 2 seconds, release smoothly for 4s
https://youtu.be/OiA1SdEBttY
Lateral shoulder raise - from standing, with (optional) light dumbells or tins of beans. Raise the arms up sideways until they are parallel with the floor, palms down, hold for 2 seconds, lower slowly (4s)
https://youtu.be/h7iFxvnuusQ
Chair squat - find a firm chair (like a dining chair). Stand in front of it and lower yourself (4s) until you feel the seat , without using your hands, hold for 2s, then stand again. Try to go steadily and smoothly. Weight in your heels, torso upright, looking ahead.

The full video (without warmup, use the separate video for that) is here:
https://youtu.be/S65GmPWA0lE

Stability 2

Straight leg dead bug - lie on your back with arms and legs straight up towards the ceiling. Lower opposite hand and leg to the floor (or half way

if you need to) then return to the starting position. Keep your torso still and your lower back pressed to the floor.
https://youtu.be/LssFq5Y5GVY
Glute bridge - Lying on your back, bend your knees and place your feet near your hips. Slowly raise your hips until you have a straight line from your shoulder to your knee, hold for 2s and slowly lower (4s).
https://youtu.be/AwHfNT-e8Cc
Single leg balance with reach - Stand on one leg in good posture, slowly reach the opposite leg, forward, to the side and back, holding for a moment in each position. Keep the pelvis and spine neutral throughout.
https://youtu.be/PxcJduiHv4o
Bench push up - Kneel in front of a low bench, table or step. Place the hands wider than shoulder width apart, thumbs level with your armpits, keep the body straight from knee to shoulder. Lower for 4s, pause for 2s, push back up.
https://youtu.be/TZ1rQo-wfM0
Band row - Sitting on the floor, feet together and straight in front of you. Loop your resistance band around your feet and hold on either side. Sitting tall, pull your elbows back, shoulder blades engaged, and row your fists towards your armpits, elbows in. Hold for 2s, release smoothly for 4s.
https://youtu.be/PSsyVsyxzbQ
Single leg scaption - standing on one leg, with optional light dumbbells (or tins of beans) in hands. Raise both arms with palms facing forwards. Your arms should be about halfway between in front of you and out to the sides. Raise for 1s, hold for 2s, lower for 4s. Change leg for second set.
https://youtu.be/w_VNrP6-jcc
Step up to balance - using an aerobics step or a stable step in your house. Step up with the right foot, bring the left knee up and hold for a second in balance, step the left foot back down then the right, repeat on the other side.
https://youtu.be/q22z5orGGQE

About the author

Claire Hunter is an Advanced Personal Trainer, Precision Nutrition Certified Coach, Bellydancer, Yogi, Doula, Powerlifter and defender of all that is awesome and has yet to realise it.

Claire is spreading the message the health and fitness should be fun, accessible and empowering for everyone.

Claire is based in Glastonbury, Somerset, surrounded by small boys and chickens. She provides online coaching and programming to people all over the world.

Find her at www.firelotusfitness.com